4 Months to Fertile

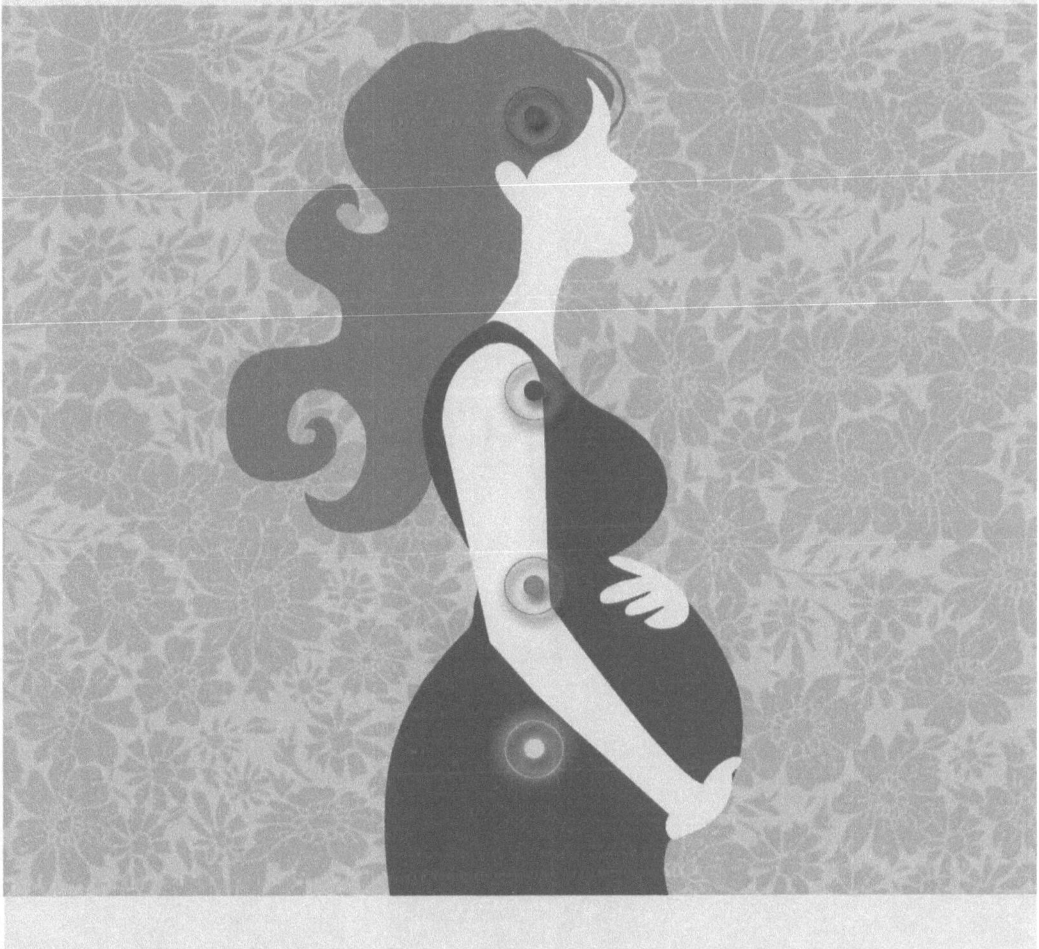

By September Burton

4 Months To Fertile

CONTENTS

4 Months To Fertile
by September Burton

www.SeptemberBurton.com

DISCLAIMER

Information provided by this e-book is meant to assist you in understanding how your reproductive system works, how fertility is perceived in the traditional Chinese medicine system and which are the factors that influence one's reproductive ability. Purpose of this publication is to help you choose the best solutions for enhancing your fertility and preparing your body for conceiving and carrying a healthy baby.

All the pieces of advice and information given in this e-book are based on reliable sources and thorough analyses, so you can trust all the recommendations given by the author. However, keep in mind that it's your responsibility to know your body and your health state and to get your physician's approval before engaging in this fertility enhancing program.

Author of this e-book is not responsible for injuries or health issues resulting from applying the recommendations in this publication. Facts provided in this e-book are accurate and considerable efforts have been made for including up-to-date information and synthesizing gathered data in an accessible manner, thus no part of this publication may be transcribed, transmitted, reproduced or translated into any language without the permission of the author.

Introduction

One of my personal favorite ways to discuss diet in relation to fertility is by relaying the story of the bees. I find bees to be absolutely fascinating little creatures. A bee colony can have millions of bees and each is genetically identical to every other one in the colony. When new eggs are laid they are all fed on a very rich substance called royal jelly for 3 days. After those first 3 days all but one are switched to honey. 1 continues to be fed royal jelly throughout her entire life.

This special bee becomes the queen. She is bigger, stronger, lives up to 20 times longer than the workers and, most importantly for our purposes, is the only fertile bee in the colony. It is nothing but her diet that sets her apart. That allows her to lay a quarter of a million eggs in her lifetime.

It therefore becomes obvious that the anatomical and functional differentiation of female bees and their reproductive ability is completely dependent on the foods they eat. It's all in their diet!

But how does this relate to fertility and pregnancy, you might ask? Pregnancy can only take place in a healthy organism, capable of producing viable eggs, of nourishing and protecting them during the various development stages.

Classical medicine says there are women who are born infertile and women who become unable to conceive due to environmental factors. But according to Dr. Deepak Chopra, world-renowned alternative medicine specialist and author of "Ageless Body, Timeless Mind", one receives an entirely new body every year, so the ability of conceiving a baby is within your control. You have the power to change your body, to fertilize your body, just like the transformation of an unfertile bee larva into a queen!

Dr. Chopra's theories, derived from the Ayurvedic system of medicine, claim that one's body can achieve what the mind believes and that one's health state can only be improved when the proper mindset is adopted. In other words, with a correct attitude towards fertility and pregnancy, you can influence your body's ability of conceiving and prepare a friendly environment for your baby-to-be.

It's therefore time for a new beginning! Commit to our fertility enhancing plan, change your mind and habits and give your body the chance to turn into its healthiest version! It will be tough and you will get discouraged, but if you keep going, you'll get there!

The first and possibly most important step is to begin to praise your body. What we praise increases, what we criticize decreases. Thank your body every day. Appreciate your body. Be amazed by your body. Accept your body, love your body and take proper care of it and it will reward you with the most fertile environment for a healthy baby to grow and develop. Take one step at a time, be patient and implement the solutions given in this book progressively. Remember, it takes around 21 days to break a habit or make a new one.

The following chapters will guide you through our fertility boosting program – make sure to read them thoroughly and to implement each recommendation and assignment as indicated, every 2-3 weeks, allowing your body to get used to its new, healthy state.

It's time to stop thinking of your body as infertile or of yourself as infertile. You are NOT infertile. Dr. Randine Lewis, author of The Infertility Cure states in her book that she no longer believes in infertility. From this moment on you are fertilizing your body! YOU are creating a new body that can easily conceive and carry a healthy baby to term!

September Burton

CHAPTER ONE

UNDERSTANDING FERTILITY

A woman's reproductive health and fertility can be affected not only by genetic endowment but also by environmental, social and physical factors. Living conditions, childhood ailments, stress, an imbalanced diet and unhealthy habits can adversely affect fertility, so there's no wonder 10-15% of all reproductive-aged couples deal with fertility problems.

The good news is one can achieve control over their body and teach the organism how to prepare for conception and pregnancy. But before discussing the strategies and methods one can use for enhancing their fertility and increasing their chances of having a baby, we'll take a quick look at the female reproductive system and try to understand how it works and why, for some couples, a little more effort is required to get it working properly.

1.1 HOW YOUR REPRODUCTIVE SYSTEM WORKS

A woman's reproductive system includes the uterus, ovaries and fallopian tubes, each of them having a specific function and being controlled by certain hormones, produced either in the brain or pituitary gland.

The number of eggs ovaries will ever release is written in one's genetic code, so even if before puberty ovaries are asleep from this point of view, once a woman enters puberty her ovaries get active and start producing higher amounts of sex hormones as well as viable eggs.

Sex hormones – estrogen and progesterone - are transported through the bloodstream and they're responsible for one's sexual development and for preparing the body to sustain fertilization and pregnancy. They regulate the menstrual cycle, ovulation and all the changes happening inside a woman's body once fertilization takes place: thickening of the uterine wall, which protects and nourishes the fertilized egg, development of the placenta, production of breast milk.

Estrogen and progesterone are also linked with the health state of one's heart, liver, bones, kidneys and many other tissues and organs. This is a very important aspect we'll discuss a little later in this chapter.

But now let's come back to fertilization and pregnancy: eggs produced by ovaries are released on a monthly basis and travel towards the uterus, through the fallopian tubes. During their journey, eggs can get fertilized when they meet the partner's sperm and once this happens, a zygote forms. This zygote will later turn into an embryo.

At birth, a girl's ovaries contain around 1,000,000 ovarian follicles from which eggs can be released but by the time she reaches puberty, this number decreases to about 400,000 ovarian follicles. From all these follicles, only one egg – called ovum - is released each month and can turn into a zygote. However, if the egg is not viable, pregnancy won't occur.

How is this egg chosen, you might ask? The process is completely random – from all ovarian follicles existing inside the ovaries, only a small number grow and develop enough to turn from primary follicles into secondary follicles, each and every month. Secondary follicles are those who can give birth to the winning egg, which will eventually become a zygote.

Remember the story about the queen bee being only fertile bee in the entire hive? This is quite a similar situation: the winning egg is the only one able to sustain pregnancy by mixing with a sperm cell. And what influences the egg's viability and the woman's fertility potential?

the

- Hormones
- Lifestyle
- Diet habits
- Genetics

If a woman's procreative ability is altered by diet and lifestyle habits, it can be restored by simply eliminating those factors that triggered the problem. Hormonal imbalances are most often caused by diet, namely excessive amounts of sugar. As far as genetics are concerned—remember, genes load the gun, but lifestyle pulls the trigger. In other words, you can control the expression of your genes.

Most complex medical treatments for fertility problems involve the so-called assisted reproductive technologies (ART), among which in-vitro fertilization (IVF) and zygote intrafallopian transfer. Success rates for IVF are around 35% for women aged 35 or less, 25% for women aged between 35 and 37, 15% for women aged 38 to 40 and less than 10% for women aged 40 and over.

How does this sound? Encouraging? Unsatisfactory? The reason these medical treatments fail in so many women is they address the effects and not the root cause of the problem. Is it really possible for an unhealthy body to produce perfectly healthy and viable eggs?

Please don't misunderstand—ART has its place. There are some couples who, due to physical deformities or other causes, know they are physically incapable of conceiving a child without help. In these cases ART is a priceless gift that modern medicine has given us. However, these couples should walk into their RE's office feeling very confident that their bodies have been properly fertilized and that they will walk out pregnant after the treatment is over. The <u>first</u> time!

Let's take a look at some interesting statistical data regarding the success rates of Chinese medicine therapy in women with fertility problems. In a study published in the journal of Complementary Therapies in Medicine, women receiving Chinese herbal medicines showed a significantly improved procreative capacity compared to those treated with classical drugs.

> Chinese medicine can double one's reproductive potential.

Success rates for the first group were around 60%, while for the control group, composed of women receiving traditional fertility treatments, these rates were around 32%.

Moreover, other studies reported a 70% pregnancy rate in women receiving Chinese medicines and acupuncture treatments. So what makes these alternative treatments so effective in restoring one's reproductive potential?

1.2 THE CHINESE MEDICINE MODEL OF FERTILITY

Chinese medicine comes with a completely different approach to fertility and this is what sets it apart from conventional medicine. This alternative system sees the human body as an inseparable whole, in which all parts are interrelated and influence each other. Balance is maintained as long as all parts function normally, but when one or more components are affected by internal or external factors, the equilibrium is altered and impairments occur.

Unlike classical medicine, the Chinese system doesn't see organs as physical structures made of tissues, but as semi-abstract concepts of functions. In this system, fertility problems are caused by deficiencies or excesses, not by altered tissues or organs, and this means the reproductive potential can be restored by simply fixing those deficiencies or excesses!

And how is this done, you might ask? The simplest answer is by maintaining the perfect harmony between Qi – which is the life force or vital energy - and blood, respectively between Yin and Yang. If you're a little confused right now, you should check the last chapter of this book, as it makes things clearer!

Now let's get back to our problem and see how these things are related to fertility. The vital energy that keeps the human body alive and normally functioning is Qi, and the Yin-Yang pairs are as follows:

- The Yin meridians of the arm are the heart, lungs and pericardium. The Yang meridians of the arm are the Intestines – small and large – and the triple warmer.

- The Yin meridians of the leg are the kidneys, liver and spleen, while the Yang meridians are the stomach, gall bladder and bladder.

Blood and Qi circulate through all these organs but when one of the meridians is hyperactive, the other becomes hypoactive so the balance is altered. A Yin deficiency – or hypofunction – triggers a Yang excess – or hyperfunction – and vice versa.

So in order for one's reproductive system to work properly, all the other organs – or meridians – have to be in equilibrium.

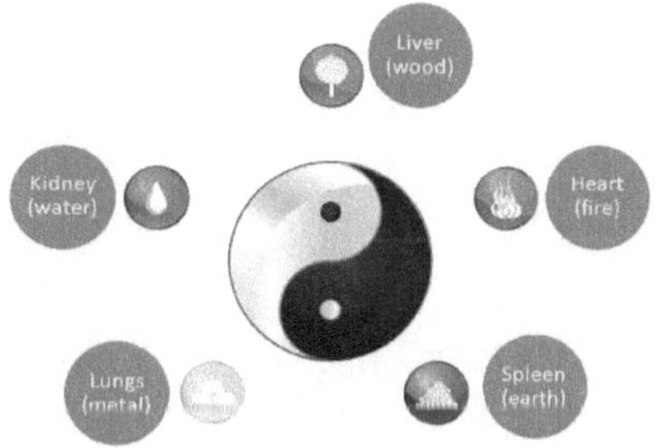

The next chapter provides an in-depth overview of the four elements that are thought to influence fertility, according to the Chinese medicine system.

CHAPTER TWO

WHAT INFLUENCES FERTILITY?

According to Chinese Medicine there are 4 organs that are specifically linked to fertility. These are the kidneys, liver, spleen, and heart. Except for the heart, all the other 3 organs associated with fertility in Chinese medicine are considered flushing organs, which is quite fascinating and perfectly logical: you must get rid of the old before you can make something new!

By restoring the balance of these meridians, one can increase their chance of conceiving as Chinese medicine is proven to be effective in:

- Improving the quality of ovules
- Regulating the hormonal levels and stimulating production of viable eggs
- Enhancing blood flow towards the uterus and increasing the thickness of uterine walls
- Decreasing stress levels and making it easier to adopt the proper mindset for conceiving
- Preventing abnormal uterine contractions
- Lessening the side effects of classical medicine therapies used in treating fertility issues
- Strengthening immunity
- Decreasing the risk of miscarriage

2.1 THE HEART

The heart is responsible for pumping blood throughout the entire body so when the circulatory function is altered, imbalances occur in all the other organs and affect all bodily processes, including procreation. This applies both in conventional and Chinese medicine; the latter system gives a clearer explanation of the link between the heart and fertility.

Ovaries receive signals from the brain, which determine the formation, growth and release of fertile ovules. However, when these signals are altered, a woman's ovulation ability is affected and therefore amenorrhea (lack of ovulation and menstruation) can occur. Obviously, without these two processes there can be no pregnancy.

All the changes taking place inside a woman's body during menstruation and ovulation can cause emotional distress, fatigue, nervousness, agitation and anxiety, insomnia, palpitations and shortness of breath. These signals may not seem related to fertility problems but they indicate an altered functioning of the circulatory system, whose main component is the heart.

Palpitations, chest pain, skin pallor, cold extremities, increased sweating and cyanotic lips and nails are other signs that indicate an obstruction of the energy flow passing through the heart. Thus, the solution to these problems and to fertility impairments caused by a blocked heart Qi is improving the health of your cardiovascular system.

The easiest way to ameliorate the functioning of your heart is to adopt a friendly diet and a healthy lifestyle, but we'll talk about these changes a little later in this book as right now we have to understand the link between spleen and infertility.

2.2 THE SPLEEN

While most people don't usually think of their spleen in relation to fertility, this organ is critical for a normal reproductive function as the main role of the spleen is to flush out old, dead red blood cells to allow for the production of new blood and immune cells.

In Chinese medicine, the spleen meridian governs most energetic processes, this organ using Qi and nutrients that are transported through the blood stream for producing new blood. Also, it is responsible for ensuring a smooth menstrual cycle, for maintaining high energy levels and for stimulating the release of certain hormones, such as those produced by the thyroid gland, which are linked with fertility as well.

An impaired spleen function triggers imbalances in hormonal levels and compromises the regeneration of blood cells, so oxygenation and nourishing of all organs is affected. The immune system becomes weaker and the reproductive system is more prone to ailments and less capable of producing viable eggs, able to generate a healthy zygote after fertilization.

So if you want to enhance your fertility, you must also pay attention to the spleen and make the needed changes in your dietary and lifestyle habits. The third chapter of this book will give you some useful pieces of advice regarding the foods you should eat or avoid for restoring your spleen's health and therefore your reproductive function.

2.3 THE KIDNEYS

In conventional medicine, kidneys are responsible for removing toxins and waste from the body, for filtering the blood, regulating its acidity and maintaining the electrolyte balance. Also, they're involved in regulating blood pressure and secreting certain hormones, which stimulate the production of red blood cells and are involved in multiple body functions, from cognition and weight regulation to fertility.

In Chinese medicine, these organs are the foundation of reproduction, development and growth. They regulate the metabolism of fluids and support a healthy sexual function, thereby maintaining youthfulness.

Kidneys are linked with a particular form of Qi, which is called the Jing Essence, in more Western terms we would call this the essence of life itself, received by each individual from their parents. Although inherited, the Jing Essence is stored in kidneys and it can be depleted through an improper diet, through excessive sexual activity, stress overload and aging.

Deficient kidneys can't store this special form of Qi properly therefore the chances of conceiving decrease. An altered kidney Qi triggers delayed menstruations, an abnormal blood flow during the menstrual period and a low sex drive. In men, it decreases the mobility of sperm cells, making it more difficult for fertilization to take place.

It's therefore obvious that in order to enhance your reproductive potential and boost your chances of conceiving a baby you must take good care of your kidneys, nourish them adequately and hydrate them properly.

2.4 THE LIVER

In conventional medicine, the liver's main functions are to store and filter the blood, to regulate the production of hormones and to ensure all metabolic processes take place normally. In Chinese medicine, the liver's main function is to ensure a smooth distribution of blood to all tissues and organs.

This organ is responsible for the production of menstrual blood as well, and is directly linked to the uterus, so it regulates ovulation and ensures a proper environment for a potential pregnancy. All the mentioned functions highlight the strong connection between liver and fertility: an unhealthy liver leads to hormonal imbalances, which alters the production and release of eggs during ovulation. If no egg is released or the produced eggs are not healthy, no pregnancy can occur.

A healthy liver on the other hand is able to dispose of old hormones more effectively and to sustain the production of new ones. Also, it ensures a normal blood flow during menstruation, when its main role is to shift the blood flow from other organs to uterus.

However, there can be days when the liver becomes so preoccupied of its function in the premenstrual period that it neglects all its other responsibilities. If this happens, smoothness of the energy flow is altered and Qi stagnations can occur anytime.

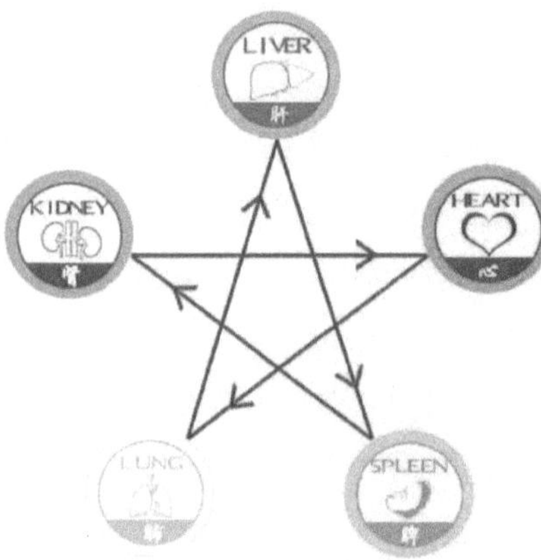

The direct consequence is a general state of malaise, manifesting through headaches and migraines, depression, cramps and breast pain, sadness and tension in the entire body. PCOS (polycystic ovary syndrome), one of the triggers of fertility impairments in conventional medicine, is often the result of an altered liver function.

As long as the channels on the liver meridian remain blocked, fertility is affected. How can this issue be solved? By improving the health of your liver.

As you can see in the picture above, liver is associated – in Chinese medicine – with the color green, so the easiest solution to restore your liver's function is to adopt a green diet. The more green foods you consume on a daily basis, the healthier your liver and entire body will become. Thereby significantly increasing your chances of conception!

But we'll talk about the proper diet for restoring your fertility in the next chapter of this book, when we'll also see what lifestyle changes one has to do in order to enhance their reproductive potential.

CHAPTER THREE

A 4 Month Plan To Enhance Your Fertility

We now know fertility can be significantly enhanced naturally, without invasive treatments, without expensive procedures and so-called miraculous kits. Chances of conceiving a baby increase when one's lifestyle and diet habits are improved and the entire body undergoes a complex detoxification, regeneration and rebalancing process.

Heart, spleen, liver, kidneys, lymphatic and reproductive systems can significantly contribute to an enhanced fertility when they're balanced so if you're ready to restore your reproductive function and your body's internal equilibrium, commit to our 4 month fertility boosting plan!

3.1 Four months to fertile

We'll first give the 8 steps that need to be followed during this 4 months plan and then take each of them and explain it for you to get an in-depth understanding of how your body will react and be transformed through these changes.

Keep in mind each of these steps needs to be implemented over a two weeks period for you to actually see and feel the results.

3.1.1 Goal 1: Kick-start your lymphatic system!

Assignment no.1: Take a sip of <u>plain</u> hot water every 10 minutes throughout the day, for 2 weeks. This first measure will pump your stagnant lymphatic system, helping your body begin to flush out toxins.

Explanation: The main role of your lymphatic system is to move the fluid out of tissues and back to the bloodstream. A stagnant lymphatic system leads to increased fluid retention and prevents your organs and tissues from being properly nourished and oxygenized.

Another consequence of lymph stagnation is an impaired immune function, which makes the body more prone to infections and ailments. Also, when your lymphatic system doesn't function as it should, toxins aren't flushed out of your body and they build up in the blood vessels and cells. Remember—out with the old to make something new.

On the other hand, a properly functioning lymphatic system moves hormones, nutrients and oxygen molecules to cells, helping them replenish and regenerate. An improper diet, lack of physical activity, environmental toxins, infections and traumas can all cause lymph stagnation.

But how is this linked with your reproductive potential, you might ask?

- Your uterus needs nutrients and oxygen just like all your other organs.
- Hormones which favor the occurrence of pregnancy are produced inside the body, so organs responsible for this function need to be properly hydrated, nourished, flushed, and oxygenized.
- A stagnant lymphatic system leads to increased stress levels and stress is proven to alter fertility.

Thus, if you want to fertilize your body and to prepare it for a pregnancy, you should first kick-start your lymphatic system by implementing measure number 1. It's your responsibility to make sure lymph keeps moving properly and all the following solutions will enhance the effects of this first measure.

One final thing to keep in mind with regard to pumping your lymphatic system is that you must pump it through exercise. Your circulatory system comes equipped with an automatic pump, your lymphatic system does not but keeping this system flowing is absolutely critical to so many aspects of health, including fertility.

So, how do you pump it? You exercise! You must get moving. And when it comes to the lymphatic system your arms are more effective at pumping it than your legs. So, make sure you are incorporating your arms into your exercise routine every day.

3.1.2 Goal 2: Cleanse your liver!

Assignment no.2: Add 1-2 glasses of green juice to your menu, every day.

Explanation: Drinking a glass of hot lemon water right after waking up or a glass of green juice helps in eliminating hormones stagnating in your liver. The healthier your liver gets, the higher the chances of conceiving become so the second step in your 4-months journey to fertility should be cleansing the liver.

This procedure is often called "fertility cleansing" and it's an easy to apply and accessible way to prepare the body for conception by flushing out old hormones and cells and making room for new ones.

But why "green juices"? In Chinese medicine, the liver is associated with the color green, as previously said, so for strengthening this organ and enhancing its function, one should consume as many green products as possible. Is this beneficial only for the liver?

Of course not - a fertility cleanse supports the health and functioning of both liver and uterus, by stimulating the elimination of toxins and excess hormones from the liver, respectively by helping the uterus get rid of stagnant blood. As a result, circulation to the uterus is improved, uterine tissues are better nourished and oxygenized so they can exert their functions in a more efficient manner.

And what toxins are we talking about? Mainly wastes left by birth control pills, pesticides and chemicals in food, cigarette smoke, alcohol and hormonal treatments. All these substances should be naturally eliminated from the organism but liver isn't always that powerful and healthy to flush all these wastes on its own.

This leads to built-up toxins, a condition which alters the liver's functioning and blood composition and decreases the body's ability of fighting pathogens. The reproductive system is affected by these aspects just like all the other organs, so it's absolutely necessary for one to cleanse the liver before attempting to get pregnant.

Opt for juices instead of smoothies as they are more effective in flushing out toxins and are more quickly absorbed into the bloodstream, nutrients from juices being assimilated in your cells within only 15 minutes.

As for foods that should be consumed for cleansing the liver and restoring its function, the list includes:

- Beets, which are very effective in flushing out hormones and preventing gallstones. Add 1-2 beets to every glass of green juice you make and drink this mixture daily. As toxins are eliminated, both your urine and feces can turn red, but please don't freak out - it's only a sign that things are being flushed. Also, keep in mind beets can throw off ovulation tests as they stimulate elimination of hormones from liver.
- Garlic and onion;
- Egg yolks, 2-4 per week;
- Cabbage;
- Broccoli;
- Cauliflower;
- Kale;

- Collard greens;
- Brussels sprouts;
- Turmeric, licorice and cinnamon;
- Rice;

Avoid processed products that are hard on your liver and opt for foods like the ones mentioned above, as they're rich in sulfur, which supports liver detoxification. Add two drops of essential lemon oil or peppermint oil to a glass of lemon water, to boost the liver's function and cleanse it from all wastes.

3.1.3 Goal 3: Adopt the proper mindset!

Assignment no.3: Begin a meditation practice. Aim for at least 10 minutes per day and do breathing exercises 2 times per day.

Explanation: YOU ARE FERTILE! YOUR BODY IS FERTILE, CAPABLE OF CONCEIVING AND CARRYING A HEALTHY BABY TO TERM! You are where your attention is. Think of yourself as fertile. Completely omit the words "infertile, and infertility" from your vocabulary. The body achieves what the mind believes. A negative attitude towards your life, body or pregnancy won't help you conceive, just like stress overload won't make you forget about your condition.

What your body needs in order to get properly prepared for conception is relaxation and a healthy mindset, a positive attitude and a high level of confidence. A daily meditation practice is the most effective way to find peace with any challenge you may be facing in life.

If you give your body the time to relax and focus on positive things, on healing, on your organs functioning at top notch, that's what your body will achieve. Focus on pregnancy, on healthy organs!

You are what you focus your attention on. Just think a little – the human body has two fundamental functioning modes - survival and reproduction. These are its two main concerns in life and unfortunately, most people live their lives in the "survival" mode, focusing only on their busy schedules, on their jobs, stressful life experiences, and on their appearance.

Survival comes first, reproduction comes second. The only solution for allowing your body to focus on its reproductive potential is, therefore, to get yourself out of the survival mode. How is this done? - Through meditation and breathing exercises.

Learn how to breathe correctly in order to oxygenate each individual cell in your body. Learn how to overcome stress overload so that your body won't waste too much energy on finding solutions to stressful situations.

Given below is an effective and fast way to bring relaxation in your daily schedule. Make sure to perform this exercise twice a day, every day, until your body gets used to it:

- Breathe in slowly through your nose for a count of 4
- Hold the breath for a count of 8
- Breathe out through your mouth for a count of 7

Repeat this for 4 breaths and try to think of each and every cell in your body plumping up with oxygen. Can't find motivation to incorporate this routine in your daily schedule? Remember stress causes inflammation and inflammation causes infertility, as well as pre-term labor once you do become pregnant. Thus, teaching your body to relax and helping it get over stressful situations is absolutely critical for conceiving and delivering a healthy baby!

3.1.4 Goal 4: Restore your kidneys' function!

Assignment no.4: Find 5 recipes you love, made of kidney-friendly foods and incorporate them in your weekly menu. Increase water intake to flush out toxins. Do this for 2 weeks, until your body gets used to the new routine.

Explanation: Kidneys being your life force, their health is very closely related to fertility. You can't get pregnant until your kidneys' function is restored and the most basic way to begin helping your kidneys is to drink plenty of fresh water daily. Aim for 2-3 liters per day.

Opt for spring water and add 2 tablespoons of unpasteurized, unfiltered apple cider vinegar to your glass of water, three times a day, to accelerate the removal of toxins from your kidneys.

Avoid soda like the plague and don't go for the cheapest vinegar found in grocery stores as the process of filtering and pasteurizing renders it worthless at best and possibly even damaging.

Besides applying these simple solutions, make sure to keep an eye on your diet and to add to your menu foods that enhance kidneys' health, sustaining toxins elimination. If you don't know which foods are considered helpful in restoring your kidneys' health, check the recommendations below:

- Burdock root, a seasonal vegetable typically found in the colder months, which looks like sticks of wood. It has a nice flavor despite its not so nice appearance. Add it to soups, stews, sautees, etc.;
- Cranberries or any other berries;
- Red bell peppers;
- Cabbage;
- Garlic;
- Onions;
- Adzuki beans;
- Apples;
- Cauliflower;
- Fish;
- Red grapes;
- Any deep purple food is going to be great for your kidneys;

These should be consumed raw, in soups, stews and sautéed veggie dishes to promote kidneys' detoxification and stimulate the removal of waste.

3.1.5 Goal 5: Revitalize your spleen!

Assignment no.5: Stop consuming processed foods and artificial sugars.

Explanation: A healthy spleen is linked with higher chances of conceiving so flushing out toxins from your spleen should be among your priorities as well. This 5th assignment should be implemented over a 2-weeks period just like the previous ones.

Start by eliminating highly processed foods and products rich in artificial sugars from your diet. Pay attention to juices, as they're often loaded with lots of substances your spleen and body don't need. Help your spleen get rid of all these unnecessary compounds and focus on enhancing your health and on having a healthy and clean spleen.

Besides limiting or completely eliminating sugars, another useful measure for cleansing your spleen is to drink hot water every 10 minutes, as previously instructed. Sugars and artificial sweeteners are a huge burden for your liver and spleen so if you can remove them from your diet, do so; but if you can't give them up completely, try switching to healthier alternatives, such as <u>green</u> stevia or raw honey (be careful with honey. Try to buy it local and be absolutely certain it is raw).

Real maple syrup, thanks to its high content of magnesium, is another healthy alternative to artificial sweeteners.

Also, make sure to adopt a diet that's spleen-friendly, including leafy green and root vegetables, carrots, barley, pumpkins, squash, parsnips, sweet potatoes, cayenne, pepper, cinnamon, nutmeg and ginger.

3.1.6 Goal 6: Eat to avoid inflammation and food intolerances!

Assignment no.6: Start reading ingredient lists thoroughly. Watch out for any vegetable oils such as soy, cottonseed, corn or canola as well as for any wheat ingredient.

Explanation: The three "foods" most Americans eat every time they sit down to eat are vegetable oils, gluten and sugar. These ingredients, present in almost all processed foods, are absolutely destroying fertility: vegetable oils are very high in omega-6 fatty acids, which can lead to inflammation when out of balance with omega-3 fatty acids.

In order for your body to stay healthy, the omega-6/3 ratio should be anywhere from 4:1 to 1:1. But with our unhealthy diets, this ratio is about 20:1 or even more! Such a low amount of omega-3 fatty acids is not enough to counter inflammatory processes triggered by excess omega-6 fatty acids. And an inflamed body is definitely not a fertile one, so if you're planning on having a baby you should try to reduce the intake of vegetable oils. Also, consider adding an omega-3 supplement to your daily routine. I recommend <u>Vital Choice</u> as they do not refine their oils.

Now let's move to sugars: it's well known that too high amounts of blood sugar throw off you your body's hormonal balance. Eliminating sugary foods from your diet is one of the easiest ways to restore your body's internal equilibrium, to decrease the risk of developing conditions that could interfere with a potential pregnancy and to keep PCOS (polycystic ovary syndrome) away. If you have a sweet tooth and need a sugary treat from time to time, stick with fruits or the sweeteners mentioned above.

As for gluten, intolerance to this substance is often the root cause of infertility in men and women alike. Gluten intolerance is linked with PCOS and PID (pelvic inflammatory disorders), both responsible for infertility. Thus, in order to enhance your reproductive potential, you should give up gluten before and during pregnancy. Gluten has been strongly linked to cases of unexplained infertility as well as to early and late miscarriage, and even stillbirth. It is also strongly linked to Autism so avoiding it during pregnancy decreases chances of Autism showing up in your child later.

But this doesn't mean switching so called "gluten free" processed foods, as these ones are often loaded with harmful ingredients that don't promote a healthy reproductive system. Giving up gluten means eliminating all products made of modern wheat, as over hybridization of these grains has led to a 300% increase in the amount of gluten found in wheat.

The right solution is to stick with ancient strains of wheat, such as kamut, spelt and einkorn, although staying away from gluten grains for good during pregnancy is even better. Reduce the intake or eliminate wheat, barley and rye from your diet and eat oatmeal in small amounts, as even if it doesn't contain gluten in itself, it's often contaminated in factories.

Besides gluten, vegetable oils, and sugar, dairy products should also be consumed in moderation and only raw, as processed dairy has been found to have negative effects on fertility. Moreover, processed dairy products consumed during pregnancy can lead to chronic ear infections in infants and small children, so unless you keep it raw, it's better to leave it alone.

3.1.7 Goal 7: Prepare your heart for pregnancy!

Assignment no.7: Add vegetables to your breakfast. They can be cooked in with eggs frittatas or just scrambled.

Explanation: A healthy heart sustains a healthy pregnancy so you should adopt a diet including lots of veggies and fruits. Still, make sure you don't neglect the importance oils, fats and animal products, as these are all good sources of omega-3 fatty acids and other nutrients needed for conceiving and delivering a healthy baby.

While many people advocate low-fat, vegetarian or vegan diets for improving your cardiovascular health, these diets aren't always the best for your other organs, which need the previously mentioned nutrients for functioning normally, regenerating and staying healthy.

So when you choose your sources of omega-3, you can opt for supplements as they don't deliver the high amounts of omega-6 fatty acids found in foods. Switch out your vegetable oils for coconut oil, ghee, and olive oil instead. If you need to prepare cooked meals, use coconut oil or ghee instead of olive oil, as this is not able to tolerate high temperatures. Olive oil is best for salads and dips.

Foods that are good for your heart include:
- Salmon and tuna
- Flaxseeds
- Oatmeal

- Kidney beans and black beans
- Almonds and walnuts
- Brown rice
- Small amounts of fermented soy such as tempe
- Berries
- Carrots
- Spinach
- Broccoli
- Sweet potatoes
- Red bell peppers
- Asparagus
- Tomatoes
- Oranges and papaya
- Squash
- Cantaloupe
- Dark chocolate (should be at least 70% cacao and watch out for added sugars)

3.1.8 Goal 8: Choose super-foods for pregnancy!

Assignment no.8: Add a smoothie made of super-foods to your daily menu.

Explanation: Certain foods are considered more beneficial for the reproductive system than others, as they stimulate the production of hormones that favor pregnancy and help the uterus prepare for hosting the baby. The number one super-food for fertility and pregnancy is camu camu berry, which can be found as powder at health food stores.

Raw cacao is also an excellent choice as it delivers an extremely high amount of magnesium, while maca is very effective in balancing progesterone levels. Goji berries, which can be found in dehydrated form in health food stores, are rich in chromium, which helps regulate blood sugar levels.

Bee products – honey, pollen or royal jelly - are known to sustain pregnancy and enhance fertility as well. Still, make sure they're raw and unfiltered when purchasing them and avoid using grocery store honey.

Following these recommendations and assignments will effectively crowd out many of the foods that are hindering fertility and will significantly improve your chances of conceiving and delivering a healthy baby.

Conclusions

We live in an era where stress reaches unimaginable levels and women put careers first, postponing pregnancy until they get to believe they're infertile and their bodies are unable to procreate. This is simply untrue. Remember—according to Dr. Chopra you get an entirely new body every single year. You can rebuild next year's model to be healthy, fertile, and much younger than this year's model.

1 in 6 couples has trouble conceiving due to unexplained infertility, although studies show couples with a history of infertility have 80% chances to procreate if they undergo fertility treatments and do the needed changes in their eating and lifestyle habits.

But we have to be aware of the fact that food isn't as nutrient rich as it once was and lots of products promoted as "healthy" are in fact harmful for our bodies. In order for a woman to fertilize her body and get pregnant, she needs to first detoxify her body and restore its internal equilibrium by rebalancing the organs that interfere with her reproductive potential.

Fortunately, this can be done by following some simple diet rules:

- Drinking more fresh water for detoxifying the liver and getting the lymphatic system moving
- Eliminating sugars, vegetable oils and gluten from their diets before and during pregnancy
- Incorporating kidney-friendly foods in their menus, for flushing out toxins and improving blood's composition and the transport of nutrients to cells
- Opting for foods rich in omega-3 fatty acids and increasing the intake of vegetables, as these improve the functioning of the cardiovascular system and sustain a healthy heart
- Eating more "super-foods" that are known to boost fertility and increase the chances of having a baby

Besides these measures, one should also try to relax, to get rid of negative thoughts and adopt a healthy mindset and a positive attitude towards pregnancy.

Believe you can, follow our plan and you'll get there!

Getting your body fertilized and preparing it for pregnancy can be a tough process so before committing to any program that claims to help you in enhancing fertility and increasing your chances to conceive a baby, you should get an in-depth understanding of this health problem.

Reading this e-book is surely an excellent way to get familiar with the functioning of your reproductive system as well as with the internal and external factors that can affect your reproductive potential and fertility. It's a very helpful step in understanding the changes that need to be done in order to restore your organism's balance and eliminate the culprits for infertility.

This e-book is meant to inform and guide you through a 4 months program that will boost your fertility and prepare a baby-friendly environment inside your body. However, given the length of this program, it's possible for you to lose motivation and feel the need of receiving more support in order to make all the changes suggested in this book.

Our 4 Months to Fertile Coaching Program is meant to assist you in overcoming the barriers that keep you from achieving a healthy, balanced and perfectly fertile body. All you need to do is follow the link above, sign up for the 4 Months to Fertile program and let us help you achieve your goal!

BONUS CHAPTER

THE CONCEPT OF QI

Qi is the Chinese concept that defines the vital energy making life possible. It's the continuous flux of energy that suffers endless transformations and generates all the things in the universe by changing its manifestation. Qi is found in solids just as it is present in fluids and gas. Without the constant movement of this vital energy life wouldn't be possible, so it's the accumulation of Qi that produces life and the dispersion of this flux that puts an end to life as we know it.

Qi cannot be seen but it's the most essential part of one's body as without it, no life activities are possible. Absolutely all substances, cells and organs in one's body are transformed and regenerated by the constant movement of this energy flux, the paths through which Qi flows being called meridians.

These meridians correspond to specific organs and they're generated and interconnected by Qi. However, in order to talk about balance or deficiencies and understand how Qi and fertility are linked, we have to define two more concepts present in Chinese medicine and these are Yin and Yang.

Meridians are divided into Yin and Yang groups, which represent opposite elements and can only be understood and exist in relation to one another. If Yin is the form, then Yang is the function and if Yin defines the material, Yang represents the immaterial. Yin and Yang form a whole: darkness can't be defined without knowing what brightness is and heaviness can't be defined without establishing what lightness is.

Yin is used for defining the substantial, material, solid and heavy, dark, cold, descending, passive and quiescent manifestations of Qi. Yang defines the amorphous, immaterial, light, hot, ascending, bright, active and hollow manifestations of Qi. However, there's no such thing as a purely Yin material and no element that's purely Yang. Yin and Yang suffer continuous transformations but their balance is maintained by Qi.